EXPLORING ENGINEERING CAREERS

Exploring BIOMEDICAL ENGINEERING Careers

Terri Dougherty

ReferencePoint Press

San Diego, CA

For more information, contact:
ReferencePoint Press, Inc.
PO Box 27779
San Diego, CA 92198
www.ReferencePointPress.com

LIBRARY OF CONGRESS CATALOGING-IN-PUBLICATION DATA

Name: Dougherty, Terri author
Title: Exploring Biomedical Engineering Careers/by Terri Dougherty.
Description: San Diego, CA : ReferencePoint Press, Inc., 2027. | Series: Exploring Engineering Careers | Includes bibliographical references and index.
Identifiers: LCCN 2026002594 (print) | LCCN 2026002595 (ebook) | ISBN 9781678212827 library binding | ISBN 9781678212834 ebook
Subjects: LCSH: Biomedical engineering--Vocational guidance | Engineering--Vocational guidance | Professions | Occupations
Classification: LCC R856.2 .D68 2027 (print) | LCC R856.2 (ebook)
LC record available at https://lccn.loc.gov/2026002594
LC ebook record available at https://lccn.loc.gov/2026002595

CONTENTS

Biomedical Engineer at a Glance

Working Conditions

Hospitals, manufacturing settings, research facilities.

Licensing

Professional Engineer license needed for advancement after working in the field for four or more years; Certified Biomedical Equipment Technician and Certified Clinical Engineer licenses available for specialized areas

Personal Qualities

- Analytical skills
- Communication skills
- Creativity
- Math skills
- Problem-solving
- Research skills

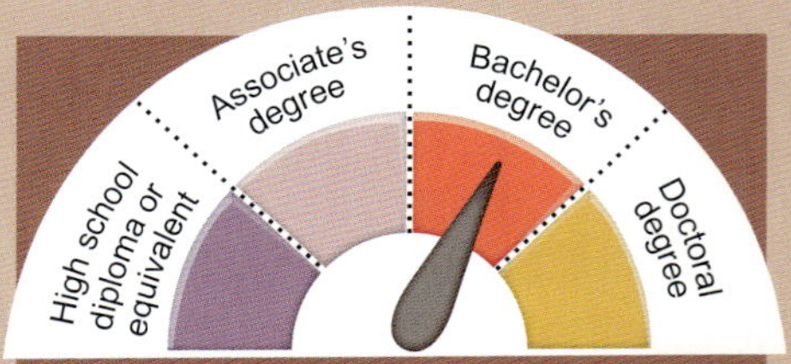

Minimum Educational Requirements

Bachelor of science in biomedical engineering or a related engineering field

Pay

$106,950 median salary

Future Job Outlook

Growth through 2034

5%

22,200

Number of jobs

Bureau of Labor Statistics, ""Bioengineers and Biomedical Engineers," *Occupational Outlook Handbook*, August 28, 2025. www.bls.gov.

Biomedical Engineers Make a Difference

Biomedical engineering student Hope Gibbons uses data from magnetic resonance imaging brain scans to create a 3-D model of a brain artery. She and her fellow students are working with their professor to find a way to predict whether a bulge in an artery, called an aneurysm, is likely to rupture and cause a stroke, brain damage, or even death. To do this, they use computer modeling and data analytics in hopes of saving the lives of future patients.

Engineering Feats Are All Around

Like all engineers, Gibbons uses math and science to solve real-world problems to benefit humanity. Looking around, it does not take long for anyone to see the impact that engineers make in the world. Smartphones, televisions, laptops, airplanes, roads, and medical equipment all get better because of work done by engineers. Applying knowledge and creativity, engineers push boundaries that bring advancements in construction, medical care, and technology. They conduct tests and inspections to ensure that products, equipment, and systems are safe and reliable. The results of their work make a tangible difference in people's lives every day. While all engineers apply mathematical and scientific concepts to technical problems and use critical thinking to design solutions, the field of engineering is varied. Civil engineers concentrate on structures and roads and make sure they are designed soundly. Mechanical engineers design equipment and machinery, while electrical engineers create and test electrical equipment. Environmental engineers tackle problems involving pollution, erosion, and flooding, as well as air, water, and soil issues. Computer engineers work with technology, creating devices, systems, and software, and chemical engineers improve products and the way they are made.

In biomedical engineering, engineering principles interconnect with the world of medicine. These engineers combine an understanding of engineering with knowledge of anatomy, physiology, medicine, and biology, and their work leads to advances in patient care, health, and well-being. One biomedical engineer might contemplate a better way of detecting cancer. Another might work to create a prosthetic hand that acts and feels natural. Still another might examine the best methods to use patient data to fight disease and develop personalized treatments for those who get ill.

Developing Lifesaving Treatments and Tools

Thanks to the work of biomedical engineers, patients routinely benefit from medical innovations. The health care field now has dialysis to remove fluid and waste from kidneys when they fail, artificial heart valves to replace those that are not working properly, pacemakers that keep the heart beating the way it should, and advanced imaging technology that provides a detailed look at the inside of the body and helps doctors more accurately diagnose and treat disease.

The possibilities and potential of biomedical engineering initially surprised Namita Khajanchi, who works with DNA as a lab technician and has a master's degree in biomedical engineering from the University of Wisconsin. She recalls:

> While I was studying chemistry at Amherst College, I spent a year at Dartmouth College and took a few engineering classes. One of the classes was a bioengineering course where I learned how scientists can introduce specific

> genes into cells to change how the cells work. . . . I was amazed that we could use engineering principles to manipulate living systems. That experience opened my eyes to an entire field I hadn't considered before . . . and I fell in love with it, so I decided to apply to graduate school for biomedical engineering.[1]

Biomedical engineers have the opportunity to develop lifesaving tools, treatments, and procedures, and the effect they have on people's lives brings meaning to their work. Alana Niximacco's interest in biomedical engineering was spurred by health problems her mother experienced. "Seeing that there were medical devices that were helpful to her and could keep her around for us made a big impact on me wanting to go into biomedical engineering," says Niximacco, who has a biomedical engineering degree from the Milwaukee School of Engineering. "I love what I do because of the impact I can make."[2]

"I was amazed that we could use engineering principles to manipulate living systems. That experience opened my eyes to an entire field I hadn't considered before and I fell in love with it."[1]

—Namita Khajanchi, University of Wisconsin biomedical engineering graduate

A biomedical engineering degree provides the background for a broad range of job opportunities. Graduates may work in research for a medical device manufacturer or a hospital. Niximacco is a human factors engineer, ensuring that patients and medical professionals can easily and safely use the medical devices made by her company. Khajanchi works with DNA sequencing for a company in Cambridge, Massachusetts. Biomedical engineers are often part of a team that includes scientists and other engineers who work together to help improve people's lives. Their work could bring about a new cancer treatment or allow a person with spinal cord injuries to regain movement. "With a career as broad as biomedical engineering, you can go into so many different specialties," Niximacco notes. "Having so much different knowledge coming out of school is really exciting."[3]

CHAPTER ONE

What Does a Biomedical Engineer Do?

For years Emily Graczyk of Case Western University and her fellow researchers have worked to make an artificial hand feel like part of the body by providing users with a sense of touch. Their work has led to a prosthetic hand that communicates with a person's nervous system. When electrodes implanted in the arm detect muscle movement, signals are relayed from the prosthetic hand to the brain. This brings sensations that the body interprets as physical touch.

Biomedical researchers at the University of Wisconsin-Madison are studying the intricacies of cells as they look for ways to make cancer treatments more effective. A team including biomedical engineering student Sophie Mancha used a microscopic imaging technique to learn more about how cancer moves away from the main tumor and spreads to other parts of the body. Their discoveries about the movement of cell clusters may help explain why pancreatic cancer can be aggressive and challenging to treat.

The work of biomedical engineers like Mancha and Graczyk leads to advances in patient care and medical devices as well as improvements in disease prevention, diagnosis, and treatment. Biomedical engineers apply engineering principles to health care, and their findings improve the lives of patients who benefit from discoveries that make their daily lives easier and more fulfilling. The artificial limb created by Graczyk and her team not only allows people to do more, it makes them more self-confident. "Having a sense of touch improves so many different aspects involved in quality of life," Graczyk notes, "including the sense of connectedness to loved ones, self-sufficiency, self-image and social interaction."[4] For Mancha, the cancer cell study's findings had a personal connection. Her grandfather died of pancreatic cancer when she was in high school, and she notes that the team's discoveries highlight the continued need for research that can lead to targeted treatments.

Solving Problems

Whether they are working with medical devices or conducting research, the work of a biomedical engineer begins with a problem that needs to be solved. This could relate to the way a procedure is done, medicine is delivered, or a disease is diagnosed. It could also involve simplifying or enhancing a medical device or making it in a more cost-effective way.

For Matt Knoespel and Phil Terrien, solving a problem meant finding a better way to care for newborns with serious heart defects. When they were students at the University of Wisconsin, an associate professor of cardiology turned to the school's biomedical engineering design program when looking for an easier way to monitor heart rhythm in infant patients. He wanted a simple way to get continuous information about how the young patient's heart was performing. Knoespel, Terrien, and their team created a device that sent cardiac signals to a bedside monitor and could be connected to a pacemaker. After graduation, they cofounded a medical device company and continued to work on refining the product. They added safety features and made other enhancements needed for US Food and Drug Administration (FDA) approval. That approval was granted four years after their college design project was completed, and their company now creates heart monitoring equipment used by children's hospitals nationwide.

Designing Devices

Biomedical engineers also create and improve devices—such as exoskeletons, wheelchairs, and prosthetics—that assist with mobility. When teenager Maggie Eggleston was looking for a brace that was lightweight, stable, and inconspicuous, she turned to University of Wisconsin–Madison biomedical engineering students for help. She has a type of muscular dystrophy that affects the muscles in the face, shoulders, and upper arms. But specifically, she needed to address the difficulty she experiences in lifting the front of her right foot.

> **"The main objective [of our muscle brace] was to find something that was functional but also very sleek-looking."[5]**
>
> —Lucy Hockerman, biomedical engineering student

A team of students took on the task of creating a device that met her needs. They used computer-aided design software, 3-D printing equipment, motion capture technology, and a testing system to create a prototype. The completed device uses an adjustable compression sock to support the foot and a brace made of carbon-fiber plastic to keep the ankle from rolling. "The main objective was to find something that was functional but also very sleek-looking and can kind of pass as almost an athletic brace,"[5] explains student Lucy Hockerman.

Working at the Cellular Level

Sometimes the solutions created by biomedical engineers cannot be seen with the human eye. These professionals work at a microscopic level to develop new treatments and therapies that can help the body do a better job of fighting diseases such as cancer. They might look for a new way to identify cancer biomarkers, such as genes or proteins, in blood. They could also edit genes to treat disease or work on injectable stem cell cultures that repair damaged tissue.

Researchers in a Columbia University biomedical engineering lab are using bacteria and a virus to infect and destroy cancer cells. Their work pairs a bacteria's ability to get to the interior of

Healing Animals, Helping People

Dustin Williams, an adjunct professor in biomedical engineering at the University of Utah, is looking for a better way to treat bone infections in people. Along the way he is helping injured animals like Major.

Major is a terrier whose back leg was severely injured when he was attacked by another dog. A serious infection set in, but the wound healed thanks to a pouch filled with antibiotics that was placed directly on the wound. The refillable pouch was developed by Williams and Nicholas Ashton, research assistant professor of orthopedic surgery at the university.

Antibiotics seep through the pouch's membrane, easily bringing them right to the wound site. "Cats hate taking pills," Williams notes. "But with the pouch, you can just empty it and refill it every day and the cat doesn't even care. And the wound heals up like a champ."

Seeing how the pouch works for animals provides vital information that the researchers can use when modifying the system to one day treat people with serious injuries and infections. "The rates of infection for orthopedic procedures have gone unchanged for 70 years," says Williams, who is also a professor of orthopedic surgery at the university. "The need is there. My goal is to heal people."

Quoted in University of Utah Health, "How Biomedical Innovation Is Healing Animals to Help People," December 9, 2025. https://uofuhealth.utah.edu.

tumors with the virus's ability to infect and get rid of the cancer cells. Using bacteria to deliver the virus gets around the body's immune system, which would ordinarily fight the cancer-killing virus. "The bacteria act as an invisibility cloak, hiding the virus from circulating antibodies, and ferrying the virus to where it is needed,"[6] explains Zakary S. Singer, a researcher in the lab of Tal Danino, biomedical engineering associate professor at Columbia University who leads the project. Inside the tumor, the bacteria self-destruct and release the virus, which has been modified so it cannot spread in healthy tissue. More work needs to be done, the researchers note, because the virus is prone to mutations, and more safeguards need to be evaluated. However, their discoveries could lead to improvements in other treatments.

Biomedical engineers also use a technique called gene editing to make precise changes within a cell. Krishanu Saha, professor of biomedical engineering at the University of Wisconsin–Madison, uses a gene-editing enzyme to create medicines that can be used to treat inherited conditions such as sickle-cell anemia and Huntington's disease. The gene-editing enzyme acts like molecular scissors, entering a cell's nucleus and cutting a slice of DNA. Once its work is done, the gene-editing enzyme will ideally disappear so that it does not cause damage. Getting rid of it is not easy, however, and Saha and his team are looking for ways to turn off the gene-editing activity. To do this, they are using a drug that would trigger a cell to gobble up the gene-editing enzyme after its work is done.

Designing with Data

Data is often used by biomedical engineers as they look for ways to improve treatments. At the Massachusetts Institute of Technology (MIT), researchers are getting help from artificial intelligence (AI) to design antibiotics that can fight drug-resistant infections.

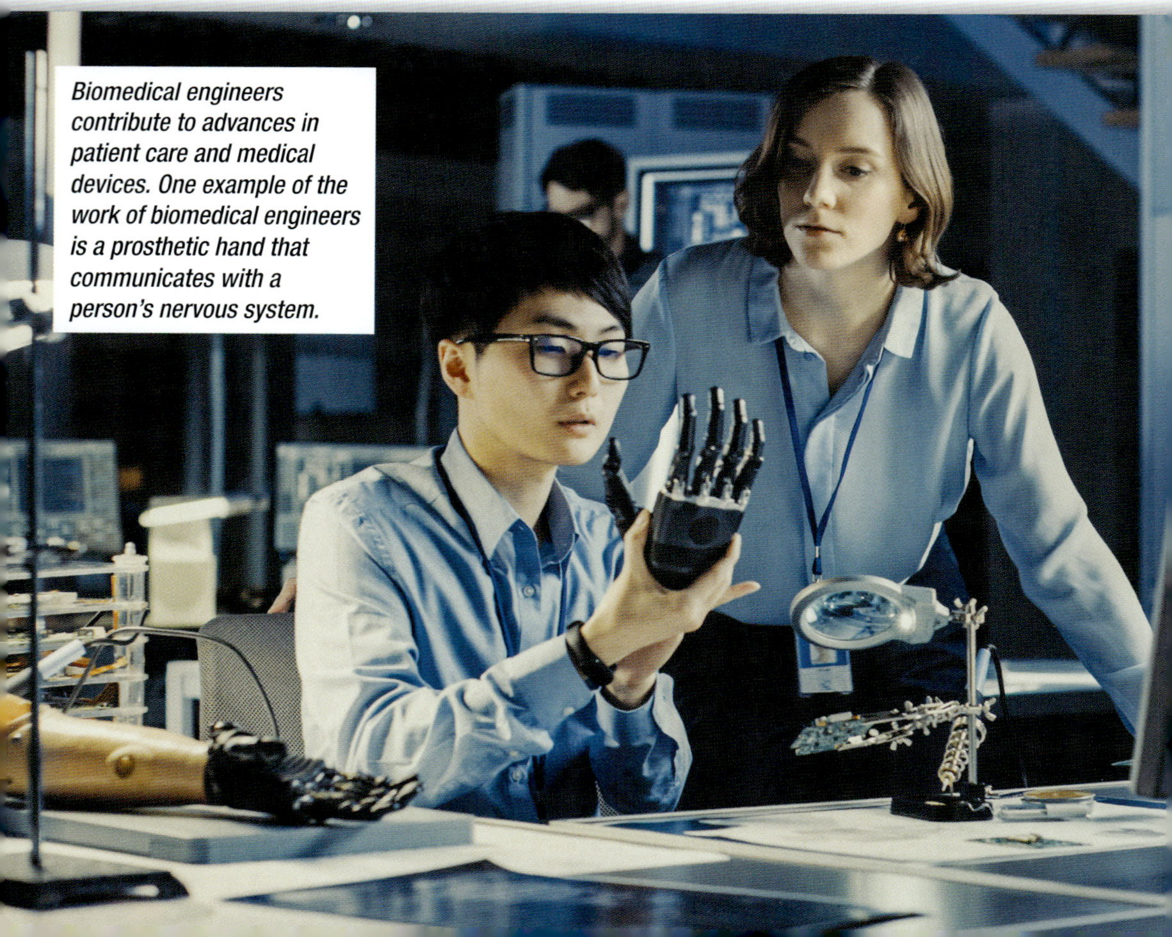

Biomedical engineers contribute to advances in patient care and medical devices. One example of the work of biomedical engineers is a prosthetic hand that communicates with a person's nervous system.

Using generative AI, the team searches chemical compound libraries to determine whether overlooked compounds exhibit any antimicrobial properties that might be useful in overcoming drug resistance. One team is even using AI to test infection-fighting treatments by combining chemical fragments into new compounds that have not yet been discovered or do not exist. Overall, generative AI designed more than 36 million possible compounds that were then screened for their effectiveness.

> **"Our work shows the power of AI from a drug design standpoint."[7]**
>
> —James Collins, professor of biological engineering at the Massachusetts Institute of Technology

The MIT researchers found that the top compounds had a structure that was different from existing antibiotics, and all seemed to use a new way to disrupt the cell membranes of bacteria. "We're excited about the new possibilities that this project opens up for antibiotics development," says James Collins, the study's senior author and a professor of biological engineering at MIT. "Our work shows the power of AI from a drug design standpoint, and enables us to exploit much larger chemical spaces that were previously inaccessible."[7]

Improving Diagnosis and Treatment

Research conducted by biomedical engineers can also lead to improvements in medical equipment, such as magnetic resonance imaging (MRI) and computed tomography (CT) scanning machines that provide a look inside the body. At the Duke University School of Medicine, Dan Ma, an associate professor in biomedical engineering, is working on MRI technology that detects tumors and abnormalities faster than current equipment.

She is working with a medical imaging company to bring an improved solution to market that scans for patterns that identify abnormal tissues. "It's similar to human fingerprints at a crime scene," Ma explains. "You may get just partial fingerprints. But you can still find the suspect because you have a powerful algorithm to extract information from those imperfect fingerprints."[8]

The technology Ma is working on has the potential to find hidden trouble spots and improve the way conditions such as brain tumors, breast cancer, prostate cancer, and epilepsy are detected and treated. While her project is distinctly focused on medical imaging, it has something in common with the work of all biomedical engineers. Whether they are improving medical equipment, using data, or conducting research on the cellular level, biomedical engineers have the same goal: to improve human health.

CHAPTER TWO

How Do You Become a Biomedical Engineer?

Sarah Scheerer's interest in biomedical engineering was sparked during a biology course in high school, when her teacher approached biology as a mechanical system. "I hadn't thought about the biological processes as a series of steps," she recalls. "This is so cool. I want to do THAT."[9] To reach her goal, she applied for the biomedical engineering program at Virginia Tech University and was accepted.

A four-year bachelor's degree program in biomedical engineering, like the one Scheerer completed, is a common way to begin a career in biomedical engineering. Biomedical engineers may also get a degree in a related field, such as math, science, or chemistry. Another option is a degree in another engineering discipline, such as mechanical or electrical engineering. A student with a strong interest in mechanical engineering may opt for a degree in biomechanics, a subset of biomedical engineering that applies mechanical engineering principles to the body's systems.

A master's degree, which requires one to two additional years of study, is often needed for leadership roles or jobs in research and development. Because Scheerer hopes to get a job in research and development, she entered a biodesign master's degree program at Virginia Tech after graduating. A master's degree program allows a student to focus on a specialized area of interest such as biomedical imaging, biomechanics, or biomaterials engineering. It can also help prepare individuals to launch their own company.

Earning a Doctorate

A doctoral degree (PhD) is needed to conduct research or teach at a university. Mike Schnieders, a professor of biomedical engineering at the University of Iowa, notes:

> Many of the cutting-edge product development teams at biomedical engineering companies or pharmaceutical companies are led by someone who's earned a PhD, because the process of earning a doctoral degree embeds in you the thinking and problem-solving skills you need to work on complex four- to five-year projects. . . . You learn not only how to think about a project strategically, but also how to write about it.[10]

"The process of earning a doctoral degree embeds in you the thinking and problem-solving skills you need to work on complex four- to five-year projects."[10]

—Mike Schnieders, professor of biomedical engineering at the University of Iowa

A doctoral degree can also be required for leadership roles in companies that focus on research in specific areas, such as tissue engineering, biological data analysis, cancer technologies, or the development of advanced therapeutic devices. Students studying for a doctorate take advanced courses, conduct original research on a specific topic, write a dissertation, and defend their findings. It typically takes five to seven years to complete a doctoral degree.

Building a Foundation in Math, Science, and Engineering

Students who are interested in biomedical engineering careers can take classes that prepare them to look at problems from an engineering and a biological perspective. High school students can prepare for a college biomedical engineering program by taking classes focused on science and math. These include chemistry, biology, and physics, as well as geometry, trigonometry, and

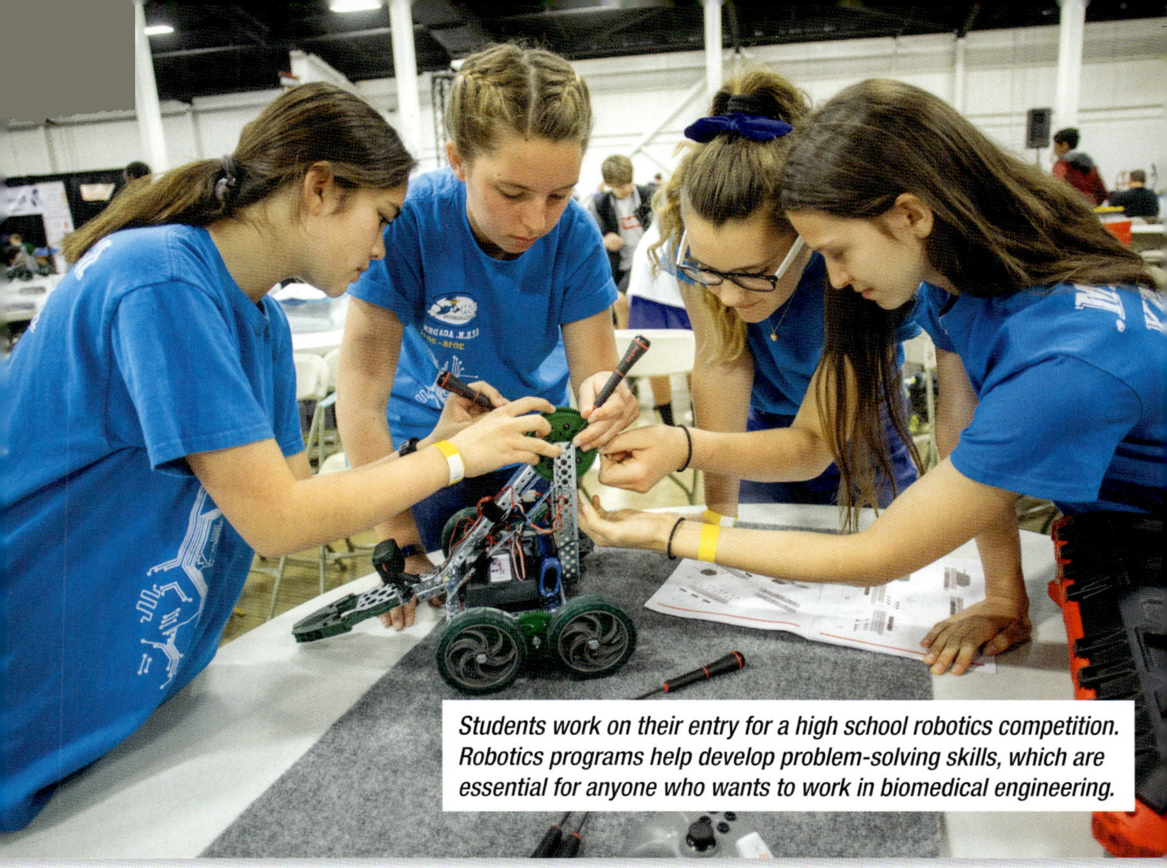

Students work on their entry for a high school robotics competition. Robotics programs help develop problem-solving skills, which are essential for anyone who wants to work in biomedical engineering.

calculus. Classes in drafting, mechanical drawing, and computer programming are also helpful. Participating in activities outside the classroom, such as robotics teams and science fairs, can help develop problem-solving skills.

College curriculums vary from school to school, but like most engineers, biomedical engineers take many math-based courses. They include calculus, differential equations, statistics, and physics. These courses provide a foundation for higher-level classes that use math to analyze complex systems and address real-world problems. Leon Zhao, who graduated from Brown University with a biomedical engineering degree, found that he used many of the concepts he learned in calculus and differential equations in his engineering courses.

Chemistry courses are also required, and Zhao recalls that one of his most difficult classes during freshman year was inorganic chemistry. While it included some high school chemistry, it added theoretical components, he notes. Other common foundational classes for biomedical engineering students include organic chemistry, anatomy, physiology, and molecular biology.

Biomedical engineering students also take engineering fundamentals courses, and one of Zhao's favorite classes was called dynamics and vibrations. It involved studying the principles of motion in mechanical systems and applying them in a practical setting. Engineering-focused classes can also include electrical circuits, instrumentation design, and fluid mechanics. Other typical classes include biomaterials, medical imaging, and biomedical devices. Zhao notes that in his biomechanics course, the math formulas and analysis methods he learned were applied in a biomedical context. "For example, we were using a stress matrix to represent the stresses on a bone,"[11] he explains.

A biomedical engineering degree also gives students the opportunity to take specialized courses that appeal to their interests. This can include classes in robotics, data science, neurobiology, or medical electronics, as well as thermodynamics, nanomedicine, and orthopedic biomechanics.

Project-Based Work

A significant part of a biomedical engineer's education involves applying learned concepts to real-world projects. Laura Wenger, who received a bachelor's degree in biomechanics from Virginia Tech, worked on several projects during her sophomore year. They included devising a medication management system for dementia patients and creating a urine collection device. She was also part of a design team that worked on a device for dialysis patients. The projects gave Wenger the opportunity to learn from her peers and broaden her knowledge base. "I really enjoy researching and digging into areas I don't really know about,"[12] she comments.

Biomedical engineering students often complete a degree with a capstone course or design project during their senior year. This also typically involves working on a team to design a device

Too Much Focus on Grades?

Josh Atcher has seen it happen: College freshmen enrolled in biomedical engineering classes who struggle to get the good grades they were used to getting in high school. This is not a reason to panic, however. The coursework is challenging, but tutoring can help and other assistance is available. "Once they get a handle on time management and adjust their study habits, they usually see the GPA rebound in their sophomore, junior, senior years," notes Atcher, director of academic advising and student support at the University of Iowa College of Engineering.

If Laura Wenger could go back in time and give herself a piece of advice, she would tell herself to stop worrying so much about her grades. She found that success in biomedical engineering classes can mean concentrating on what the course is about rather than only on a grade point average. "It may sound counter-intuitive, but when I gave up fighting for As and focused on learning the content, I learned so much more," comments Wenger, who received a bachelor's degree in biomechanics from Virginia Tech. "My grades improved too."

Quoted in University of Iowa, "Biomedical Engineering Degree Requirements: What You'll Need, from Start to Finish," 2026. https://uiowa.edu.

Quoted in Virginia Tech Biomedical Engineering and Mechanics, "Class of 2023: BEAM Outstanding Senior Laura Wenger," 2026. https://beam.vt.edu.

or solve a problem faced in the medical field. This hands-on project gives students the opportunity to see how their skills make a difference in people's lives. Scheerer was part of a team that redesigned an IV pole, which holds bags of intravenous fluids that are administered to hospital patients. She found it fulfilling to be involved in a project that made nurses' jobs easier.

Internships

Biomedical engineering students also gain valuable experience through internships and co-ops. During a semester or over the summer months, student interns may work in a hospital or lab, or with a medical design firm or another organization. This offers the opportunity to learn from people working in the field and see how skills can be applied in a real-world setting.

An internship can also spark ideas. Scheerer identified the need for IV pole improvements during a summer internship before her senior year. During her internship she interacted with surgeons and nurses, and while shadowing a nurse she saw that IV poles could be better designed.

Career insights can emerge from internships as well. During a six-week summer internship between her sophomore and junior years, Wenger worked with three other students on a biodesign project that aimed to create a wearable device to help people with lymphedema, a chronic condition that leads to swelling in the arms or legs. Over the next two years, the team worked to fine-tune the device, ultimately taking second place in a competition for medical devices that have commercial potential.

The internship showed Wenger that she enjoyed working with patients. After graduating from Virginia Tech, she went on to study for a master's degree in prosthetics and orthotics at the University of Texas Southwestern Medical Center. "I knew I wanted to work individually with patients, to actually see them," she says. "It was important to me and I wouldn't have known that if I hadn't been involved with the lymphedema project."[13]

Performing Lab Research

Biomedical engineering students can also get hands-on experience by working in university research labs. Universities often con-

Overcoming a Setback

Matt Knoespel and Phil Terrien did not get to work on their first-choice project in a biomedical engineering design class at the University of Wisconsin–Madison, and that setback had a profound impact on their careers.

They and three teammates reluctantly chose another project and created a device prototype that could monitor an infant's heartbeat. The device won the Tong Biomedical Design Award, the top award in the university's biomedical engineer design program. It also led them to found Atrility Medical, a medical device company that received a Wisconsin Innovation Award in 2022. "It turned out to be a life-changing selection that was thrust upon us, to some degree," says Knoespel. "When doors close, new ones open, and sometimes you don't expect that."

Quoted in Tom Ziemer, "Biomedical Engineering Alums Find Rhythm at Design Program Spinoff," University of Wisconsin–Madison College of Engineering, February 13, 2023. https://engineering.wisc.edu.

duct research that leads to breakthroughs in the medical field, such as better ways to deliver medication or advances in medical instrument design.

> "Working in the lab helped me understand my coursework better because I could relate it to real-life applications."[14]
>
> —Carolynn Que, Michigan Technological University biomedical engineering graduate

Working in an instructor's lab helped Carolynn Que see how her courses applied to work done in the field. While a student at Michigan Technological University, she focused on creating solutions that combined solvents and polymers to create nanofibers. The goal was to come up with technology that would speed up the healing process of wounds, such and burns as diabetic foot ulcers. "Working in the lab helped me understand my coursework better because I could relate it to real-life applications,"[14] says Que, who received bachelor's and master's degrees in biomedical engineering.

Degree Opportunities

Colleges and universities with biomedical engineering majors may be accredited by ABET (formerly known as the Accreditation Board for Engineering and Technology). The organization assesses schools offering degrees in science, technology, engineering, and mathematics fields, and schools accredited by ABET meet the organization's standards.

A biomedical engineering degree can lead to a career in a variety of areas, from research to product design to health care. A student may decide to concentrate on biomaterials, cell and tissue engineering, medical imaging, or another aspect of the field. It is very common not to have a specific area of specialization in mind upon entering college, and schools typically offer students the opportunity to explore a broad range of options.

Students who do have a strong interest in a certain aspect of biomedical engineering should keep that in mind when exploring colleges and universities. "If you're more inclined to computer science, make sure your program incorporates coding classes. Interested in product development? Make sure there are courses in computer-aided design or access to 3D printing," advises Kelsey Lyons, who graduated from the University of Iowa with a biomedical engineering degree and then went on to study at the Georgetown University School of Medicine. "Biomedical engineering encompasses a broad range of interests, so make sure the school has the resources to support the track that interests you,"[15] says Lyons.

CHAPTER THREE

What Skills and Personal Qualities Are Needed Most—and Why?

Julie Liu, an associate professor of chemical and biomedical engineering at Purdue University, had a question. She and her team wondered whether it was possible for a surgical wound to heal without staples or stitches. Could glue-like material allow healing to happen without the patient experiencing pain, getting an infection, or going back to the doctor for removal?

Finding the answer required technical knowledge of biology, chemistry, and materials science, but it also involved soft skills—personal and social skills that allow people to cooperate and communicate effectively. Liu's team had to collaborate with scientists from other disciplines and work through setbacks. They persisted as the research stretched over years. The work they did led to a breakthrough sealant that they patented, but they were not done refining it yet. When seeking researchers to continue the work on surgical adhesives, Liu looked for highly motivated independent researchers with a variety of abilities that included technical knowledge as well as excellent written and communication skills.

Biomedical engineers like those on Liu's team certainly need to have a solid understanding of math and science, but they also need skills that enable them to work effectively as part of a team and connect with people from outside their area of expertise. In addition, they need to have the discipline and fortitude to think critically, pay attention to detail, and not give up when challenges arise. As they work toward a solution to a complex medical problem, biomedical researchers need to be creative and inventive, merging technical knowledge with unique insights and experiences to come up with practical solutions.

Technical Skills

Math and science skills provide the foundation for a biomedical researcher's work. Biomedical engineers use advanced math to design solutions, analyze how they are working, and troubleshoot problems that arise. An understanding of calculus, differential equations, and statistics helps them comprehend the intricacies of the medical devices they work with and manage the complexities of the problems they are looking to unravel.

Because their work involves designing solutions that impact the human body, they also need to understand how the body works. This requires a working knowledge of biology and chemistry.

Having the Courage to Take a Chance

Carolynn Que was keenly interested in the work being done in an instructor's lab at Michigan Technological University, but before she could sharpen her skills in the lab she had to be brave.

Que, who received bachelor's and master's degrees in biomedical engineering from the university, became interested in the lab during a tour. She hesitated to ask to join the instructor's research group, however, because of her grades. "I chickened out for two months," she recalls. "Then I happened to run into her in the hallway one day. It was just the two of us and I mustered some courage, counted to three and blurted out the question. I flushed immediately thinking about how clumsy it sounded and patiently awaited her refusal. To my surprise, it never came. Instead she casually agreed to meet with me to discuss a potential project."

Through her work in the lab, Que honed her problem-solving skills and learned something about herself. "It is okay not to know everything," she notes. "Working in the lab restored my confidence in myself and helped me realize GPA [grade point average] is just a number."

Carolynn Que, "My Story: Carolynn Que, MTUengineer," *Biomedical Engineering News* (blog), Michigan Technological University, October 6, 2023. https://blogs.mtu.edu.

A sound grasp of engineering principles is also critical, as biomedical engineers apply these principles to the human body. Knowledge of fluid analysis and structural analysis might be used to design a new artificial heart valve or prosthetic limb or analyze fluid movement in the brain. Concepts of electrical engineering can be used in designing electroencephalogram (EEG) machines that monitor brain activity or imaging systems such as MRI machines and CT scanners that show what is going on inside the body. Knowledge of chemical engineering can lead to a targeted drug delivery system or tissues engineered in a lab. Familiarity with biomaterials could result in the development of a new material that can be safely used in the human body.

Computer Programming

To analyze data, biomedical engineers use software programs and computer programming skills. Computer-aided design and computer-aided manufacturing tools are used to create models of human tissue, implants, and medical devices. Biomedical engineers may also use a programming platform such as MATLAB to do data analysis and image processing. During a summer research internship for incoming college freshmen at the University of Arizona, Kapil Inguva used MATLAB code to capture biological information from MRI data. He used the biological information to create virtual models that could be used to analyze differences in the flow of cerebrospinal fluid and brain activity. The goal was to find areas of the brain that could show a link between fluid levels and brain health, which could lead to insights into diseases such as Alzheimer's disease.

Artificial intelligence is also used by biomedical engineering researchers, since it can analyze massive amounts of data quickly. This can bring innovations that lead to breakthroughs in disease diagnosis and individualized treatment plans for patients. At the University of Texas at Austin, biomedical engineering professor Pengyu Ren works with computational biomolecular engineering. Researchers in his lab use AI in their development of new drugs and drug delivery methods, and he has cofounded a company that uses supercomputers and software to do computations that lead to the discovery of new drugs. University of Texas at Austin associate professor Ed Castillo uses computational biomedical engineering in medical imaging research. His work involves the use of mathematical modeling, simulations, data analysis, and algorithms. This can lead to a deeper understanding of how the body's processes work, both normally and when impacted by disease, on the molecular, cellular, tissue, and organ levels.

Curiosity and Creativity

Curiosity and creativity are also assets for biomedical engineers, because a research project typically begins with a question. Biomedical engineers wonder why things work the way they do or whether an idea could lead to an improved way to deliver medical care or treatment. They put creativity to work as they devise an original way to improve a product or solve a problem, often considering innovative and inventive solutions.

When searching for a better way to close surgical wounds, Liu's team looked in an unusual area: bodies of water. They wanted a surgical seal that would work in a wet environment, and they turned to natural glues for inspiration. To better understand how this could work, Liu looked at how sandcastle worms and mussels were able to stick to objects underwater. Their ability to produce a protein that had adhesive strength, even when wet, was the key, and researchers mimicked this type of adhesion when developing a new bonding material.

Communication

Expertise from researchers in many fields is required to tackle medical problems like the one Liu and her team are working on. Because these professionals often collaborate, biomedical engineers need excellent communication skills and the ability to work as part of a team. While biomedical engineers may work independently to complete their portion of a project, they need to communicate with peers and others outside of their area of expertise to share important information. To achieve a goal, they may work with scientists, engineers, physicians, patent attorneys, physical therapists, business professionals, and technical writers.

Biomedical engineers also need to explain what they are working on and make their breakthroughs understandable to an audience not familiar with scientific terminology. For example, Liu spoke of the ability of undersea mussels to attach themselves to rocks to describe the type of adhesive qualities she was hoping to copy. Her research proposal said:

> Look to the seas and you will find creatures such as mussels, barnacles, and oysters sticking themselves to wet rocks. Man-made adhesives, by contrast, fail miserably when tasked with wet adhesion. Consequently, we rely upon painful sutures, staples, and screws to repair damage from injuries or surgical procedures. Our laboratories are working together in developing a series of new adhesives to connect tissues when surrounded by blood.[16]

By comparing the goal of her work to an oyster's natural ability to stick to a wet rock, Liu's complex project was presented in a way that most audiences could understand.

Problem-Solving and Perseverance

A problem that needs to be solved, such as the quest for a better surgical suture, is at the heart of a biomedical researcher's work. Biomedical researchers need to be adept at problem-solving yet must recognize that solutions do not arise in days, weeks, or even months. Their work takes years and could be refined throughout their entire career. Liu's team published their first paper on their surgical suture breakthrough in 2017, and almost a decade later, researchers were continuing to improve the product.

Biomedical researchers must persist through challenges as they use trial and error to reach solutions. It can be challenging

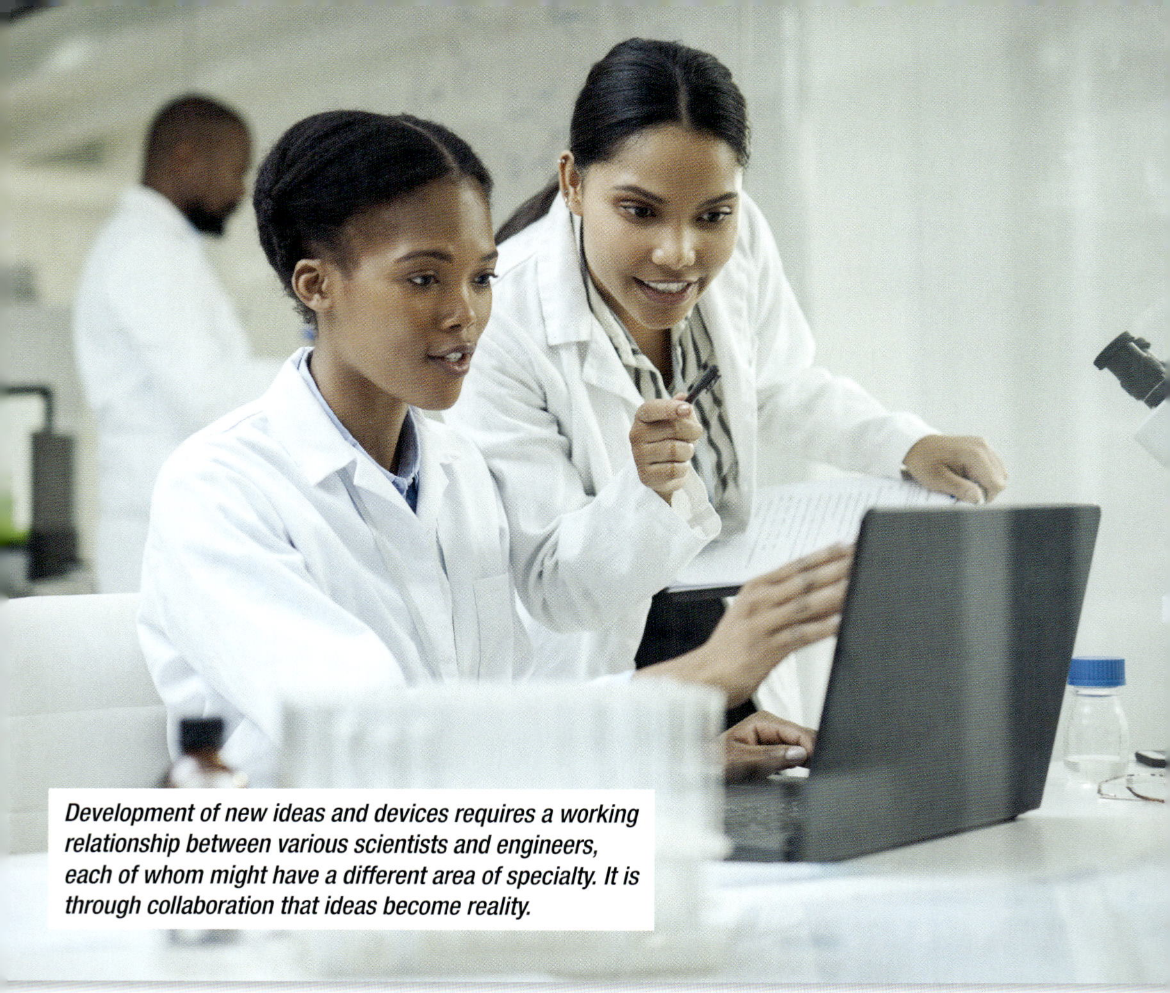

Development of new ideas and devices requires a working relationship between various scientists and engineers, each of whom might have a different area of specialty. It is through collaboration that ideas become reality.

to work through failures and setbacks, and biomedical engineers need to understand how to cope with unexpected results and deal with frustration without giving up. While a student at Michigan Technological University, Carolynn Que worked in an instructor's lab. One of the things she learned was to accept the outcome of an experiment, even when she did not like what she saw. "Things are what they are," she says, "and I will find a use for them or modify experiments to achieve better outcomes."[17]

> **"Things are what they are and I will find a use for them or modify experiments to achieve better outcomes."[17]**
>
> —Carolyn Que, Michigan Technological University biomedical engineering graduate

When designing and testing the viability of a product, treatment, or device, biomedical engineers need to be precise and accurate. They must thoroughly understand a problem and how it impacts a patient or medical professional, and this requires analytical thinking. Biomedical engineers analyze complex data and think critically about the results to determine how to move forward. "Applying what we learn comes down to being able to synthesize a lot of information to come up with solutions,"[18] notes University of Iowa biomedical engineering graduate Kelsey Lyons.

"Applying what we learn comes down to being able to synthesize a lot of information to come up with solutions."[18]

—Kelsey Lyons, University of Iowa biomedical engineering graduate

What Is It like to Work as a Biomedical Engineer?

Georgia Gadsby works on new medical devices, and the work she is doing on any given day depends on where a product is in the creation process. The process begins with the construction of a prototype that Gadsby, a product development engineer, then tests in a lab. The product also goes through a clinical trial before she presents the results to physicians and hospitals. "One of the most rewarding things about a career in biomedical engineering is being able to see the products that you release in the market and the benefits they have on the population they're treating,"[19] she notes.

> "One of the most rewarding things about a career in biomedical engineering is being able to see the products that you release in the market and the benefits they have on the population they're treating."[19]
>
> —Georgia Gadsby, product development engineer

Alana Niximacco makes sure those who use medical devices can do so safely and efficiently. Niximacco has a job in human factors and usability research at a medical device company. She works with products such as infusion pumps, respiratory devices, and laparoscopic surgery tools. She reviews designs and regularly communicates with engineers and others in her company about everything from product design to packaging features. In addition, she and her team test the products with those who will use them. "A group of intended users could be asked to complete a task so the researcher can evaluate what can be understood and what isn't intuitive about the design, and what errors might be made,"[20] she explains.

Where Do Biomedical Engineers Work?

Biomedical engineers work in industry, research, and health care, and the day-to-day work they do depends on the organization they work for as well as their individual role. Those who work for a medical device company, like Gadsby and Niximacco, work in various phases of product development as they focus on bringing innovative products to medical professionals and patients. A biomedical engineer whose job is geared toward the manufacturing of a medical device may work with a quality assurance team to test a product and make sure it meets standards before it is sent to a hospital or clinic for use. A biomedical engineer focusing on research could work in a lab at a university, medical facility, or medical research company. Another career option is to work for a government agency and ensure that medical products meet safety and regulatory standards.

The Bureau of Labor Statistics notes that 22 percent of biomedical engineers and bioengineers work in research and development in the areas of physical, engineering, and life sciences. Medical equipment and supplies manufacturers employ 14 percent of biomedical engineers, while 10 percent work for professional and commercial equipment and supplies wholesale companies. Another 10 percent work in health care and social assistance, and the final 4 percent work in engineering services.

A Typical Day

Biomedical engineers collaborate with other scientists and engineers as they develop products and work toward innovations in medical care, but they also spend time working independently. They may meet with their project team or connect with professionals using their products to get feedback to learn what is

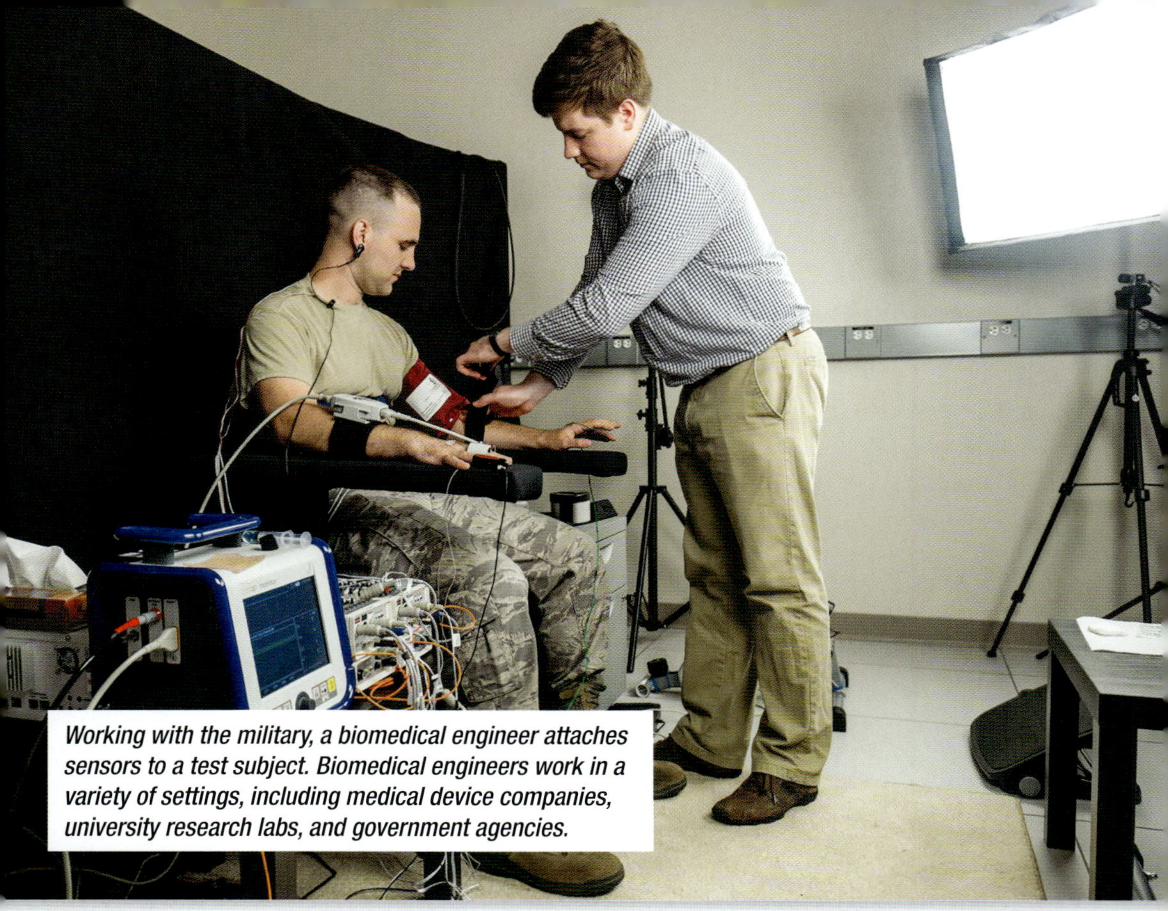

Working with the military, a biomedical engineer attaches sensors to a test subject. Biomedical engineers work in a variety of settings, including medical device companies, university research labs, and government agencies.

working and where improvements can be made. A biomedical engineer might also spend time testing a prototype or device to make sure it meets quality standards.

Creative problem-solving and troubleshooting are part of a day's work. Gadsby not only creates prototypes of the medical devices she is designing, she also has to find a way to test them. To do this she uses equipment set up in her company's lab, where she also builds the parts she needs. In addition, she comes up with creative ways to see whether a device will work. To test a respiratory device, for example, she might ask a healthy person to pedal an exercise bike to simulate the experience of a patient who is having difficulty breathing. "In the biomedical specialization you're kind of building everything," she says. "You're building the testing equipment that you use to investigate your parameters as well as products that you use in the market."[21]

Documentation is also important in the process of bringing innovations to market. Before a medical device can be sold, it needs regulatory approval from the FDA. To grant approval, the agency must be assured that the device is safe and has been thoroughly analyzed and tested. Biomedical engineers may analyze the product, gather data from clinical trials, and write an assessment that is submitted to the agency for review.

Salary

A biomedical engineer's salary depends on employer, duties, and experience. An entry-level biomedical engineering job will pay less, while those that require more experience will have a higher salary. The lowest-paid 10 percent of biomedical engineers earn less than $71,860 annually, while the highest-paid 10 percent earn more than $165,060, according to the Bureau of Labor Statistics.

Biomedical engineers earn competitive salaries. The median annual wage for biomedical engineers and bioengineers is $106,950, according to the bureau. This is more than twice as much as the median pay of $49,500 for all occupations. It is slightly higher than the $106,070 median salary for all engineers.

When it comes to finding a job in biomedical engineering, location also matters. Some states have a higher concentration of jobs in the health care, biotech, or medical device industries. The University of Iowa lists California, Washington, Minnesota, Texas, Indiana, Ohio, Pennsylvania, New York, Massachusetts, and Connecticut as the ten states with the highest employment for biomedical engineers.

When looking at the various types of biomedical engineering occupations, the Bureau of Labor Statistics reveals that those working in engineering services have the highest pay, at a median of $125,010 annually. Those working for professional and commercial equipment and supplies merchant wholesalers make $122,520 a year, while those working in research and development in the physical, engineering, and life sciences earn

$108,990 annually. Biomedical engineers working in medical equipment and supplies manufacturing make $103,020 a year, and the median annual pay for those in health care and social assistance is $95,440.

Work Hours

Biomedical engineers typically work full time and may need to put in overtime to finish a project. A job in biomedical engineering requires dedication and hard work but also leaves room for other activities. Niximacco works forty to forty-five hours a week when not conducting testing and about sixty hours a week when testing is underway. Earlier in her career she put in eighty hours a week during testing weeks, but she now uses consulting teams to help run the testing to improve her work–life balance.

While many biological engineers work during the day, for some the workday begins in the evening. Lab technician Namita Khajanchi works for a company that sequences DNA, and she works at night to make sure customers get their results the next day. To get the process going, Khajanchi arrives half an hour before her 7:00 p.m. shift to get things ready in the lab. "Sometimes I need to prep samples that need to be re-run, and other times I even do some 3D printing for lab tools or parts," she says. "The main goal on my shift is to sequence the genomes of bacteria and yeast and get results back to people as quickly as possible."[22]

"The main goal on my shift is to sequence the genomes of bacteria and yeast and get results back to people as quickly as possible."[22]

—Namita Khajanchi, lab technician

To begin the process of sequencing DNA, she loads a robotic device with materials like pipette tips and reagents that are used to create a reaction. She must make sure the robot is working properly. If something does not look right, her engineering side kicks in, and she troubleshoots by checking calibrations and fixing issues. After the reactions are initiated, Khajanchi then labels the samples and transfers them to another machine to perform the sequencing. "After that, it's all about monitoring the run, checking for problems, and making sure the data is high quality and will reach our customer on time,"[23] she says.

Maintaining Wellness

Keeping on top of projects can be mentally demanding, so biomedical engineers have to find ways to stay focused and energized. For Khajanchi every day is a little different, depending on the number and quality of samples and the tools that are being used. She says this keeps her job challenging and exciting. Working in the evening can get lonely, since her coworkers leave several hours into her shift, but if she needs to bounce ideas off someone or troubleshoot a problem, she can call coworkers in other locations who are still working.

Taking part in favorite activities during non-work hours can also relieve stress and support well-being. In her free time, Niximacco enjoys sewing, crafting, and going on walks with her family and their dog. Although Khajanchi works from 7:00 p.m. to 3:00 a.m. from Tuesday through Friday and from about 3:00

Biomedical Engineering Jobs That Demand a Broad Range of Expertise

Each day brings something new for Austin Caldwell. He is a research and development engineer at a company that develops technology for diagnosing and treating medical conditions, and he feels his work offers more freedom and variety than many traditional jobs in research and development. "There are days where I have to know everything about the biological healing processes, or the difference between canine and human and other preclinical models, and how we're putting all that together," says Caldwell, who graduated from the University of Iowa with a biomedical engineering degree. "And then there are days where I need to know about the nuances of material properties and crystalline structure of nitinol. My role takes me all over the place, and I really like that."

While some biomedical engineers may focus on specific aspects of a field, those like Caldwell apply their expertise over a range of knowledge areas. That diversity can make jobs like Caldwell's more interesting even if they might be more demanding.

Quoted in University of Iowa, "Is Biomedical Engineering a Good Career?," 2026. https://uiowa.edu.

to 8:00 p.m. on Saturdays, she finds time to do what she loves to do: taking walks in the Boston Common. "People-watching is one of my favorite activities, and on nice days I bring a book and a picnic blanket so I can read and relax in the sun," she comments. "I have a great work–life balance. I make it a point to take time off when I'm feeling burnt out, and if I'm sick, my boss is very supportive and encourages me to rest so I can return at full speed."[24]

CHAPTER FIVE

Specializations and Other Job Opportunities

Alana Niximacco says she found her niche in human factors engineering and usability research because she talked too much. While a student at the Milwaukee School of Engineering, she had an internship as a systems engineer. When asked by her boss during a department meeting how things were going, she admitted she had finished the project that had been expected to take the length of her internship and was bored. "He looked at me and I thought, 'I shouldn't have said that.'" But the manager looked around the room at other leaders and said, "Who needs help?" A human factors engineer raised their hand. "I had never heard of human factors engineering, but I found good mentors and did a lot of reading and I found a career I loved,"[25] Niximacco says.

> "I had never heard of human factors engineering, but I found good mentors and did a lot of reading and I found a career I loved."[25]
>
> —Alana Niximacco, human factors engineer

A biomedical engineering degree can lead to careers in many different specializations. As a human factors engineer, Niximacco makes sure medical professionals and patients can easily understand how to use the devices made by her company. She oversees testing and ensures that the devices are safe to use. A person with a biomedical engineering degree will use the skills they learned in their studies, she notes, but may not have "biomedical engineer" in their job title.

Curious about where a biomedical engineering degree took her college classmates, she checked and found that they worked in medical device product support, project management at medical device companies, higher education doing research at universities, and manufacturing. "We all got the same degree and are mostly at medical device companies or doing research, but for those of us at medical device companies we are in such a variety of areas,"[26] she comments. Whether a biomedical engineer is interested in research, medical devices, or another facet of health care, there is most likely a specialization that will fit their interests.

Medical Device Specializations

A biomedical engineer may create medical devices that enhance people's lives, and one area of specialization is to work with bionics. This involves creating artificial limbs that are controlled by brain signals that travel along the body's nerve fibers. The devices developed by bionics engineers help improve the lives of people with disabilities. Biomechanics is another option. It involves using mechanical knowledge, information about motion, and insight into how the body's systems function to analyze injuries and develop prosthetic limbs and orthopedic implants.

Other job opportunities are found in bioinstrumentation. This field focuses on developing medical instruments or measuring devices such as fitness tracking smartwatches. An instrumentation engineer may also create new equipment or software that is used in medical device production.

A biomedical engineer's job may also focus on the design or production of medical devices. A medical device designer works to build lifesaving tools, while a manufacturing engineer creates or improves the process for making the products. A medical imaging engineer concentrates on the development of equipment—including X-ray, CT, ultrasound, and MRI machines—that helps diagnose disease and deliver pinpointed treatment. A quality engineer ensures the devices are safe to use and meet standards set by the FDA.

A biomedical engineer could also specialize in regulatory affairs, preparing and submitting technical and regulatory documents to government agencies for approval, or work for a government agency to set standards and assess new products. Abagail Bock, who got a biomedical engineering degree from Virgina Tech, is a biomedical patent examiner at the US Patent and Trademark Office. She reviews applications for electrosurgical devices that deliver energy to tissue during a medical procedure. She assesses them for novelty, patentability, and feasibility. "I work with inventors, attorneys, and other examiners to determine the best way to describe claimed inventions and improve applications for potential allowability,"[27] she explains.

Exploring Other Research Opportunities

Biomedical engineers also have many research-focused career options. A biomaterials engineer, for example, creates and tests substances that interact with the body's systems to diagnose or treat a condition. They work with natural materials as well as those

Researcher, Professor, and Company President

To bring their research to market, biomedical engineers may take on new roles. Cancer researcher Jenny Munson is a professor who directs the cancer research center at the Fralin Biomedical Research Institute at Virginia Tech. Her research team created a tool that helps show where cancer cells are hiding in the brain so they can be targeted and destroyed.

While working in academia, Munson also serves as the president of Cairina, a company that provides personalized approaches to cancer surgeries and therapies. Her university work serves as the foundation for her corporate mission. "Cairina is trying to take this to the next level," Munson says, noting that the goal is to supply surgeons and radiation oncologists with probability hot spot maps to show where more aggressive cancer treatment might be beneficial. And because cancer treatments like radiation and chemotherapy are damaging to tissues impacted by cancerous cells, identifying hot spots can help doctors spare nearby, healthier tissues from unnecessary harm.

Quoted in Matt Chittum, "Predicting Where a Deadly Brain Cancer Might Go Next," Virginia Tech News, September 9, 2025. https://news.vt.edu.

created in a lab. Their work could better enable a hip implant to form a bond with natural bone.

A biomedical engineer could also concentrate on tissue engineering, which involves growing tissues outside the body to restore, improve, or replace the body's natural tissues. At Harvard University, bioengineering doctoral student Paul Stankey is part of a team that developed a new way to use 3-D printing to create networks of interconnected blood vessels that can be placed inside human heart tissue. The team found an easier way to form the inner lining of the printed blood vessel and make it stronger to withstand the pressure of blood flow. As part of their work, the team printed a 3-D model based on a patient's artery. Their work is a step toward creating replacement organs that can be implanted into the human body.

Another option for specialization is orthopedic bioengineering, which combines tissue engineering, cell biology, and biomechanics (the way the body's muscles and bones work) to find ways to

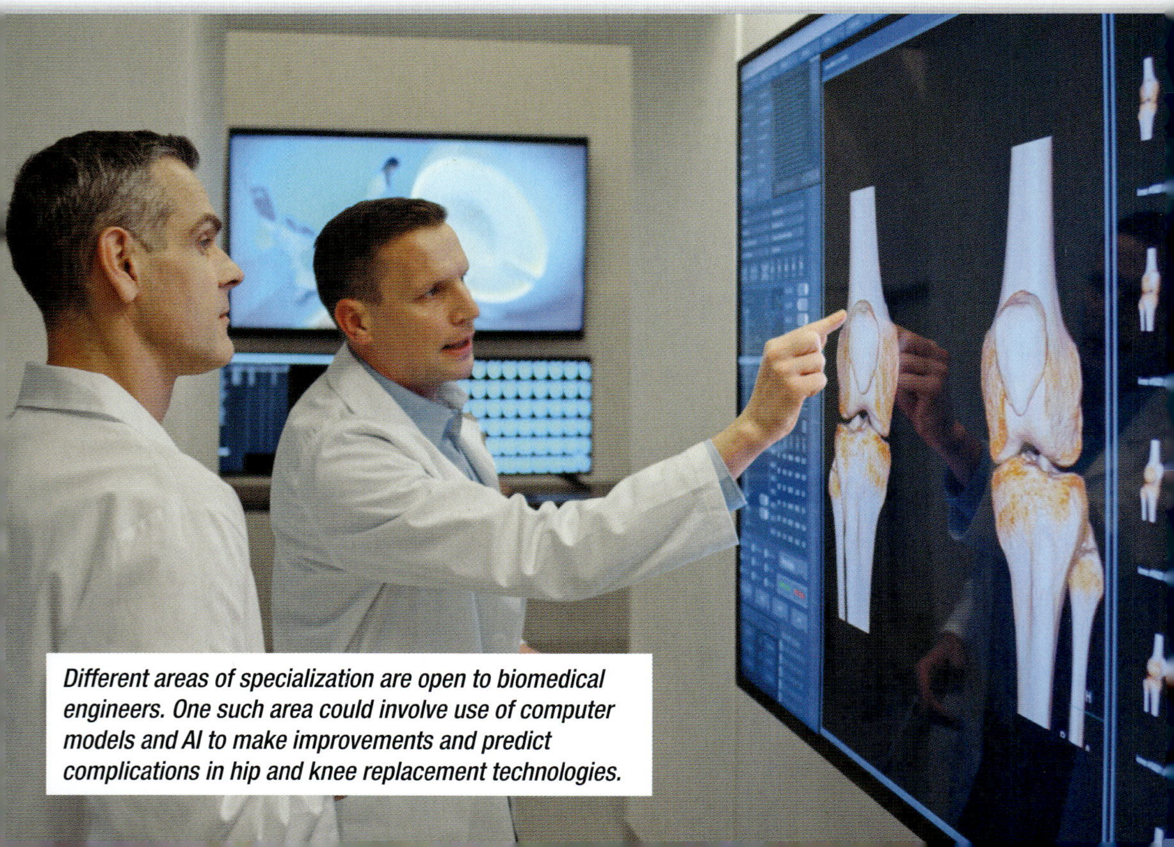

Different areas of specialization are open to biomedical engineers. One such area could involve use of computer models and AI to make improvements and predict complications in hip and knee replacement technologies.

treat musculoskeletal disease. These engineers must understand the properties of bones, muscles, and cartilage as they look for ways to promote healing. Such work might use computer models and AI to make improvements and predict complications in hip and knee replacement technologies.

Biomedical engineers could also work in the field of neural engineering, which applies engineering principles to the technology that repairs and enhances the function of the nervous system. Their work could help restore mobility to people who have been paralyzed, reduce chronic pain, and restore hearing. Advancements in the neural engineering field can lead to the development of imaging tools that are used to study the structure and function of brain tissue or improve deep brain stimulation therapy that can help people with Parkinson's disease regain control over body movements.

Moving into Management or Sales

A career in biomedical engineering research can lead to a leadership role in a company that creates products used by the medical community. John Snell began his thirty-year career in biomedical engineering doing research in the Department of Neurosurgery at the University of Virginia. After thirteen years at the university, he became chief scientist at the Focused Ultrasound Foundation, which uses precisely focused sound waves to treat tissue disorders deep inside the body. He spent more than a decade with the foundation, investigating ways to use ultrasound to treat conditions like stroke and epilepsy. He also released an ultrasound modeling system that gives scientists a look at what focused ultrasound's invisible sound waves do as they pass through the skull. He notes that his work gave him the opportunity to develop new technology and collaborate with other researchers and clinicians. Later in his career he moved into a management role with a company that used ultrasound technology to treat patients with liver tumors.

A degree in biomedical engineering can be the starting point for jobs in medical device sales, quality engineering, and consulting. Andres Calderón, who has a bachelor of science degree in mechanical engineering and a master of science and a PhD in biomedical engineering, is a forensics biomedical and biomechanical engineer. When an accident happens or someone is injured because a product does not work like it should, he uses engineering principles to explain the cause. "I have worked on cases investigating injuries such as slip, trip and falls; automobile accidents; construction related accidents; injuries from medical implants, devices, and other medical products,"[28] he explains.

Education and Advancement

While a bachelor's degree provides access to entry-level engineering jobs, a master's degree in engineering is often advised to broaden opportunities in the biomedical engineering field. A biomedical engineer interested in designing technology that assists people with disabilities may attend a two-year master's degree program in rehabilitation engineering, for example. This opens opportunities to develop communication, mobility, driving-assistance devices, and other technologies that help people with disabilities live more independently.

An advanced degree can also open the door to more opportunities in supervisory roles as well as advanced research jobs. A biomedical engineer interested in management may get a master's degree in business administration. A doctorate can lead to more research and development roles, as well as teaching, advisory, and consulting roles at a university or government organization.

Certifications and Credentials

There is no specific exam for biomedical engineers to enter their field, especially if their work falls within the private sector. However, if they hope to lead research teams, serve as the principal engineers on health care projects, or consult with the public, they must pass two exams. The first is the Fundamentals of Engineering exam, which tests both general and field-specific knowledge. The other is the Principles and Practice of Engineering exam, which tests competency and practical applications of knowledge. Passing these exams verifies that an engineer can be licensed in the United States to work for the government or with the public. An engineer can choose to take these exams even if employed in the private sector, because passing them can lead to better job opportunities and promotions.

"The field of biomedical engineering continues to evolve quickly with advances in AI, wearable tech, and personalized medicine."[29]

—Nicole Grosland, associate dean for academic programs at the University of Iowa College of Engineering

Biomedical engineers also typically join organizations such as the Biomedical Engineering Society or the National Society of Professional Engineers to stay on top of industry trends and network with other professionals. Like many careers, engineering values continued learning as ideas and applications change.

Deciding on a Path

With so many options to choose from, deciding on a career path in biomedical engineering may seem overwhelming. Nicole Grosland, associate dean for academic programs at the University of Iowa College of Engineering, advises having an open mind. "The field of biomedical engineering continues to evolve quickly with advances in AI, wearable tech, and personalized medicine," she notes. "3D bioprinting for example, is revolutionizing regenerative medicine, while digital tattoos provide a way to continuously monitor vital signs. The opportunities are endless."[29] She encourages engineers to follow their passions and interests as they explore the field.

What Does the Future Hold for Biomedical Engineers?

At one time, new drugs needed to be tested on animals before earning approval from the FDA for testing on humans in clinical trials. Thanks to the work of biomedical engineers and others, some of that preliminary testing can now be conducted with organs on chips. This technology places living human cells on glass, polymer, or silicon wafers so that researchers can replicate organ functions and study fluid movement, chemical reactions, and other cellular processes. "We're actually able to create an entire organ in one little device," notes Jason Gleghorn, an associate professor in the biomedical engineering department at the University of Delaware. "The device is about the size of two postage stamps next to each other."[30] This innovation can increase the accuracy of the testing, lower the cost, and get a drug to market more quickly.

Improvements continue to be made in the way organs on chips are created and manufactured, making them more readily available for use in research labs around the world. "We're developing bootcamps where researchers can come for two or three days" to learn how to use the device, Gleghorn notes. "If you can put it in the hands [of other scientists] and democratize the technology such that many other people can use it, you can speed the pace of innovation and you can unlock new discoveries."[31]

The drive to shorten the testing time and remove the need for animal trials points to a bright future for biomedical engineers. Their work has brought about such advancements and helped innovate in other fields, including health monitoring, prosthetics, drug delivery systems, and medical imaging technology. The potential to witness more breakthroughs creates demand for people with biomedical engineering skills and training.

> **"If you can put it in the hands [of other scientists] and democratize the technology such that many other people can use it, you can speed the pace of innovation and you can unlock new discoveries."[31]**
>
> —Jason Gleghorn, associate professor of biomedical engineering at the University of Delaware

Key Areas of Discovery

A research paper on the future of biomedical engineering, written by fifty researchers from thirty-four universities, pointed to key areas where biomedical engineering could make a significant difference in medical care and treatment. Michael Miller, senior author of the paper and professor and director of the Department of Biomedical Engineering at Johns Hopkins University, notes that work in these areas of research will impact engineering and medicine for decades.

One innovation expected to make an impact involves the use of patient data from wearable sensors. The data can be used to create avatars that help predict and prevent disease development, as well as lead to personalized care and treatment plans.

Another expected advancement involves stem cell engineering and manufacturing. A patient's own cells may one day be used in organ-on-a-chip technology, which would allow physicians to see how a patient's organs and biological systems would respond to treatment. Stem cell research may also lead to the ability to generate new tissues or organs to replace faulty ones.

The use of AI in brain research is also expected to be a key development. AI can model brain anatomy and behavior, helping scientists understand its complexities to allow for the treatment of disease.

An increased understanding of the immune system could also bring advances in treatment of diseases such as cancer and could lead to more ways to combine engineering principles with innovations in vaccines and gene editing.

A greater understanding of the human genome, the complete set of genetic information in the body, is another area of focus and could lead to disease treatments based on human cells. "These grand challenges offer unique opportunities that can transform the practice of engineering and medicine,"[32] notes Shankar Subramaniam, a bioengineering professor at the University of California, San Diego and a leader of the group of researchers who identified key biomedical research areas.

Data, AI, and Robots

As Miller and others note, AI will play a significant role in the future of biomedical engineering as it brings improvements to medical devices and treatments and reduces health care costs. It has already led to better medical imaging that can identify patterns and deviations from the norm that a human may not notice. This brings more rapid detection of disease and the opportunity to be-

Advances in Breathomics

Breath tests might become a common way to screen for cancer during routine physicals because of advancements being made by biomedical engineering researchers. At the University of Texas at Dallas, researchers are working on breath testing technology that could be used to screen for lung and esophageal cancer.

The tool uses AI to help catch cancer in the early stages, when it is easier to treat. "There is a huge amount of data provided by the breath," notes Shalini Prasad, head of the university's bioengineering department. "What is important? What is not? All of this information comes from the machine learning algorithm."

The tool is part of the emerging field of breathomics and could one day provide an easy, fast, and affordable way to test for cancer. "Eventually, this technology could be deployable in your primary care provider's office," Prasad comments. "So just as you go in for an annual physical and give an annual blood draw, you could do a breath test as well."

Quoted in Pulmonary Insights, "Biosensor Device Could Detect Lung Cancer with Breath Test," November 4, 2025. www.ampulmonary.com.

gin treatment more quickly. "There is no doubt that artificial intelligence is coming in so rapidly and it's really going to change the way we do everything," says Donald Ingber, founding director of the Wyss Institute for Biologically Inspired Engineering and a professor of bioengineering at Harvard University's School of Engineering and Applied Sciences. "If you ever have a family member who's been in the hospital and had an X-ray or a [CT] scan or MRI, it's read by radiologists, but there's no doubt it's getting so humans can't do it as good as these computers. It's not all there yet, but it's beginning."[33]

> **"There is no doubt that artificial intelligence is coming in so rapidly and it's really going to change the way we do everything."[33]**
>
> —Donald Ingber, professor of bioengineering at Harvard University's School of Engineering and Applied Sciences

Machine-based learning systems can also analyze data from heart tests and help detect abnormalities. In addition, algorithms can predict how drugs will interact with each other, which assists with the management of complex disorders. In the future, AI may help optimize drug dosages, improve robotic surgery, and lead to tailored treatment based on a person's genetic profile. It may also lead to new ways to diagnose disease. For example, it may be able to help diagnose Parkinson's disease and Alzheimer's disease using voice traits, such as tone, pitch, and cadence.

However, AI has limitations because it cannot fully grasp the context and nuances of a patient's condition. In addition, Ingber notes that it works with what data exists and therefore lacks the ability to be creative.

For Namita Khajanchi, robots are already making an impact on her work in DNA testing. Part of her job involves using a pipette to transfer a precise amount of liquid from one container to another. The tool has a plunger on the end that is pushed down to dispense the liquid, and using it repeatedly can strain the hand and nerves in the wrist. Khajanchi does not need to do the pipetting by hand, however. She has a robot do it for her. "I'm part of the future already," she comments. "The robots are very much a time saver, and keep everyone from getting carpal tunnel."[34]

Using AI to Spot Disease Triggers in the Human Genome

Yang Lu, an assistant professor of biomedical engineering at the University of Wisconsin–Madison, employs machine learning to search the human genome for markers that could signal disease. The work is complex because multiple genetic interactions could be responsible for disease progression.

"Biologists usually cannot afford to do experimental evaluation for 100 or 1,000 of these gene interactions," Lu comments. "Due to budget limitations, they can only afford, say, 10. How do we make sure the 10 we provide them with are guaranteed to be the 10 most likely to trigger the disease?" So he and his collaborators created an AI model called Diamond that helps researchers decide which results to investigate.

The AI sorts through massive amounts of genetic data to see which genes or genetic interactions could trigger a disease. But because AI can take "shortcuts" in its analysis, it is very possible that among the millions of simulated interactions, false positives occur. Diamond accounts for this and uses the AI to interrogate its own results. As Lu explains, "Diamond scores each interaction's synergistic effect and delivers a false discovery rate, a rigorous estimate of the odds that it's wrong." This allows researchers to focus on the interactions that are the more likely culprits of disease progression.

Quoted in Tom Ziemer, "New Tool Interrogates Machine Learning Models to Uncover Disease-Leading Biomarker Interactions," University of Wisconsin–Madison College of Engineering, October 8, 2025. https://engineering.wisc.edu.

She does not expect robots to take over her job, however. "Even if you have robots you always need someone to be watching them," she notes. "You can't just think that robots are going to take over all of the labor."[35]

Job Prospects

Because biomedical engineers work in several fields, from health care to research to manufacturing, and have a broad range of job options, opportunities in these fields are likely to continue to expand. The Bureau of Labor Statistics expects employment for biomedical engineers and bioengineers to grow by 5 percent through 2034. This is faster than the average growth of 3 percent for all occupations. The bureau expects an average of thirteen hundred job openings to be posted each year for biomedical engineers.

Growth in the field is due in part to the demand for biomedical devices such as hip and knee replacements. There is also greater public awareness of advances in medicine, making it likely that people will look for biomedical solutions to health problems. Finally, job openings will also occur when people retire or move to different occupations, allowing new workers with new ideas to drive growth in the field.

Advancements in technology and breakthroughs in treatment make this an exciting time to study biomedical engineering. "Innovations in the form of multi-scale sensors and devices, creation of humanoid avatars and the development of exceptionally realistic predictive models driven by AI can radically change our lifestyles and response to pathologies," Subramaniam notes. "Institutions can revolutionize education in biomedical and engineering, training the greatest minds to engage in the most important problem of all times—human health."[36]

SOURCE NOTES

Introduction: Biomedical Engineers Make a Difference

1. Namita Khajanchi, interview by the author, December 8, 2025.
2. Alana Niximacco, interview by the author, December 5, 2025.
3. Niximacco, interview.

Chapter One: What Does a Biomedical Engineer Do?

4. Quoted in Case Western Reserve University, "New Clinical Trial to Test Sensory Prostheses for People with Upper-Limb Loss," Newswise, September 4, 2025. www.newswise.com.
5. Quoted in Tom Ziemer, "BME Students Step Forward to Help Teen with Muscular Dystrophy," University of Wisconsin–Madison College of Engineering, May 19, 2025. https://engineering.wisc.edu.
6. Quoted in Inside Precision Medicine, "Virus Cloaked in Bacteria Kills Tumor Cells from Within," August 15, 2025. www.insideprecisionmedicine.com.
7. Quoted in Genetic Engineering and Biotechnology News, "AI-Designed Molecules Show Potent Activity Against Resistant Bacteria," August 14, 2025. www.genengnews.com.
8. Quoted in Angela Spivey, "Mission: A Faster, Better MRI," Duke University School of Medicine, August 27, 2025. https://medschool.duke.edu.

Chapter Two: How Do You Become a Biomedical Engineer?

9. Quoted in Michelle Darby, "Class of 2024: Sarah Scheerer Named Outstanding Senior for Biomedical Engineering and Mechanics," Virginia Tech News, May 9, 2024. https://news.vt.edu.
10. Quoted in University of Iowa, "Is a PhD in Biomedical Engineering Worth It?," 2026. https://uiowa.edu.
11. Leon Zhao, *My Entire Biomedical Engineering Degree in 16 Minutes*, YouTube, June 18, 2022. www.youtube.com/watch?v=7kR8X0AcV5s.
12. Quoted in Virginia Tech Biomedical Engineering and Mechanics, "Class of 2023: BEAM Outstanding Senior Laura Wagner," 2026. https://beam.vt.edu.

13. Quoted in Virginia Tech Biomedical Engineering and Mechanics, "Class of 2023."
14. Carolynn Que, "My Story: Carolynn Que, MTUengineer," *Biomedical Engineering News* (blog), Michigan Technological University, October 6, 2023. https://blogs.mtu.edu.
15. Quoted in University of Iowa, "Which College Is Best for Biomedical Engineering?," 2026. https://uiowa.edu.

Chapter Three: What Skills and Personal Qualities Are Needed Most—and Why?

16. Quoted in Purdue University College of Engineering, "Bioinspired Materials for Surgical Adhesive or Sealant Applications," September 12, 2025. https://engineering.purdue.edu.
17. Que, "My Story."
18. Quoted in University of Iowa, "Biomedical Engineering Degree Requirements: What You'll Need from Start to Finish," 2026. https://uiowa.edu.

Chapter Four: What Is It like to Work as a Biomedical Engineer?

19. Quoted in Tahatu Career Navigator, *This Is What a Day as a Biomedical Engineer Looks Like*, YouTube, November 20, 2025. www.youtube.com/watch?v=SgBcANVG4oQ.
20. Niximacco, interview.
21. Quoted in Tahatu Career Navigator, *This Is What a Day as a Biomedical Engineer Looks Like.*
22. Khajanchi, interview.
23. Khajanchi, interview.
24. Khajanchi, interview.

Chapter Five: Specializations and Other Job Opportunities

25. Niximacco, interview.
26. Niximacco, interview.
27. Abigail Bock, "Class of '22: Biomedical Patent Examiner at the U.S. Patent and Trademark Office," Virginia Tech College of Engineering, 2026. https://eng.vt.edu.
28. Andres Calderón, "What Is the Difference Between Biomechanical and Biomedical Engineering?," Consulting Engineers & Scientists, Inc., May 14, 2021. https://ces-experts.com.
29. Quoted in University of Iowa, "Biomedical Engineering Degree Jobs: Diverse Skills Fit a Wide Range of Career Paths," 2026. https://uiowa.edu.

Chapter Six: What Does the Future Hold for Biomedical Engineers?

30. Quoted in University of Delaware, *Innovation at UD: Jason Gleghorn*, YouTube, September 30, 2025. www.youtube.com/watch?v=3fk7c0uFdWQ.
31. Quoted in University of Delaware, *Innovation at UD*.
32. Quoted in Cornell Chronicle, "Consortium Identifies 5 Grand Challenges in Biomedical Engineering," March 20, 2024. https://news.cornell.edu.
33. Quoted in Museum of Science, *What Is the Future of Engineering with Bioengineering Pioneer Donald E Ingber*, May 11, 2024. www.youtube.com/watch?v=iEVOCD5AVr8.
34. Khajanchi, interview.
35. Khajanchi, interview.
36. Quoted in Cornell Chronicle, "Consortium Identifies 5 Grand Challenges in Biomedical Engineering."

INTERVIEW WITH A BIOMEDICAL ENGINEER

Alexis Fiechtner is a biomedical engineer at ATEC Spine in San Diego, California. ATEC makes medical devices used in spinal surgeries. She has worked at this company for three years. She answered questions about her career by email.

Q: Why did you become a biomedical engineer?

A: I discovered I wanted to become a biomedical engineering in 7th grade when I was diagnosed with a bone deformity called "miserable malalignment." Instead of my femurs and tibias growing straight like most people's, mine grew twisted at an angle. When I hit a growth spurt, the pain around my knees became overwhelming, and I eventually needed surgery.

During the surgery, my surgeons cut and re-aligned both of my shin bones so they could grow straight again. Recovery was long; I spent months in casts and a wheelchair. I then used a walker, crutches, and finally walking boots. The surgery was very successful. I had a record-breaking fast recovery and was back to playing basketball in no time.

My inspiration to become a biomedical engineer didn't just come from that experience. After surgery, my surgeon told me he had designed a special tool specifically for my surgery. He had requested it to be made a few months prior and showed it to me after the surgery.

I was shocked; I had no idea that people made medical devices. I immediately knew that I wanted to do that, too—I wanted to design devices that could help someone the way mine helped me.

That experience inspired me to become a biomedical engineer and still motivates me to do my best work every day.

Q: What does your typical workday look like?

A: Most days, I am doing a lot of 3D modeling in SolidWorks [a computer-aided engineering software]. I spend a big chunk of time working through designs and adjusting them. About 70 percent of my day is spent doing modeling.

The other portions of my day could be spent doing a couple things:

I have meetings with our marketing, regulatory, and quality teams to make sure everything we're creating is on the right track. Our marketing team shares what surgeons need from our devices. Regulatory ensures we're following FDA requirements. Quality keeps us in check with internal processes and standards so our devices stay consistent and reliable.

I'm frequently in our cadaver lab, where surgeons practice procedures using our prototypes. I watch how the devices perform, answer questions, and take notes on their feedback. After labs, I'll iterate on [rework] my designs to improve the next version.

Other days, I'm in the machine shop building simple prototypes, or in the test lab with our testing team putting devices through forces and stresses similar to what they'd experience in a patient's spine.

Q: What do you like most about your job?

A: I love the early stages of working through a challenge, the brainstorming, the sketching, the calculations, the 3D modeling. It's very exciting to have the opportunity to create something completely new and knowing it comes from your own ideas and creativity.

What makes it even more meaningful is that every problem is related to real people. The things I design are meant to help someone, to make a procedure safer, or to make a patient's life better. Knowing that I can have a direct impact on someone's life is incredibly fulfilling, and it motivates me to create the best medical devices I can.

Q: What do you like least about your job?

A: In biomedical engineering, everything we create will ultimately be used by, on, or for people, which means that safety is a top priority. To make sure of that, we have to abide by strict FDA regulations. Everything must be documented, from design choices to testing, and materials. It's not the fun, hands-on part of the job, but it is essential.

Q: What personal qualities do you find most valuable for this type of engineering work?

A: One of the most valuable qualities in biomedical engineering is the ability to find interest in the fine details, A lot of this work requires spending a large amount of time focused on a single problem, so having a curiosity and genuine desire to dive deep into figuring out how things work is incredibly helpful.

Creativity is another essential quality. Engineering is frequently associated with math and science, but the best solutions usually come from thinking out of the box. Being able to take suggestions from surgeons for designs and turn them into something real, with solid engineering calculations to back it up, takes a lot of creativity.

Q: What is the best way to prepare for this type of engineering job?

A: The best thing you could do is learn 3D modeling early, especially through classes in programs like SolidWorks. We use this software or similar software in our daily lives as biomedical engineers, and it's one of the most important skills in the engineering industry. Math and science classes are also important. Understanding materials and how they interact, forces and how they move objects, and all the basic physics of motions and structure are fundamentals that appear every day when designing medical devices, even if we don't consciously realize it.

Q: What advice do you have for students who might be interested in a career as a biomedical engineer?

A: A great place to start is by taking an anatomy and physiology course. It can help identify whether you're interested in biomedical engineering specifically or engineering in general. You can succeed in this field without loving medicine, but having a passion for understanding how the body works definitely helps.

My final advice would be to work hard and pay attention in school. Understanding how something works, the math behind it, the science of how it was made, and the physics of motion, are all really important parts of being able to successfully design a medical device for yourself someday.

American Institute for Medical and Biological Engineering (AIMBE)
https://aimbe.org
The AIMBE website provides information about the organization's advocacy efforts in support of biomedical research. The Milestones of Innovation in the student section offers a look at advancements in biomedical engineering since the 1950s. In the Fellowbook News section, articles about research being done by members are highlighted.

Biomedical Engineering Society
www.bmes.org
This organization's website provides information about the profession. The communities section offers the opportunity to join special interest groups on topics such as medical devices and cellular and molecular bioengineering. The *Office Hours* podcast offers insights into innovations and timely topics. In addition, the site provides information about membership and student chapters.

IEEE
www.ieee.org
The website for the IEEE provides information about the global community for technology professionals. It provides a look at events, conferences, and fellowship opportunities. It also includes special reports and insights into innovations in technology.

IEEE *Pulse*
www.embs.org/pulse
The website for the magazine of the IEEE Engineering and Medicine Biology Society offers a look at issues biomedical engineers are currently exploring. Topics include AI and

machine learning, genetics, precision medicine, neural engineering, and engineering ethics. The career corner provides information about mentoring programs.

Navigate the Circuit
https://navigate.aimbe.org
An overview of a career in biomedical engineering is featured on this website from the American Institute for Medical and Biological Engineering. The site includes interviews with bioengineers and a look at biomedical engineering history. It also provides information about career pathways and tools for success.

INDEX

PICTURE CREDITS

Cover: belushi/Shutterstock

12: Gorodenkoff/Shutterstock

17: Spencer Grant/ZUMAPRESS/Newscom

28: Peopleimages/Shutterstock

32: Military Collection/Alamy Images

40: simonkr/iStock

ABOUT THE AUTHOR

Terri Dougherty has written more than one hundred books for children and young adults. She loves exploring new areas and has written about a variety of topics. She lives in Appleton, Wisconsin, with her husband, Denis. They enjoy hiking, biking, and traveling, especially visiting their three children.